FERTILITY BOOSTING SMOOTHIES FOR COUPLES

Harmonizing Health and Hope: A Flavorful Odyssey for Couples Navigating the Path to Parenthood

Melinda Blevins

TABLE OF CONTENT

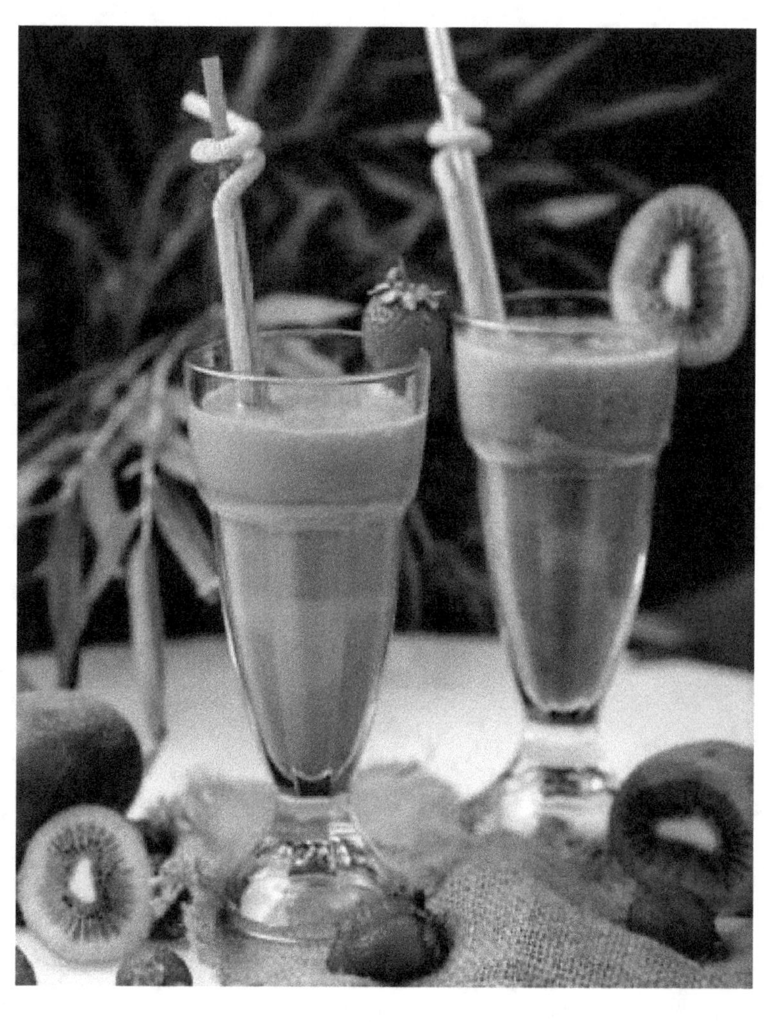

CHAPTER ONE

Introduction

Meet Sam and Sarah, a tenacious couple on a life-changing journey to embrace the joys of parenthood. They came to a fork in the road when faced with the delicate issues of fertility. It was at this critical juncture that they decided to take charge of their reproductive journey, looking for answers outside the box.

In their search for a comprehensive approach to improving reproductive health, Sam and Sarah discovered a very simple yet profoundly powerful solution: fertility-boosting smoothies. These nutrient-dense beverages, which are high in key vitamins and minerals, quickly became the foundation of their fertility-boosting strategy. The transformational impacts were not only physical; they also refreshed their spirits and strengthened their emotional well-being.

Sam and Sarah's story is not unique; rather, it serves as a model for many other couples facing comparable circumstances. Infertility, a very personal and often isolated affliction, can have an emotional, physical, and social impact. However, it is during this trial period that the potential of nutrition and lifestyle decisions to impact fertility is revealed.

This in-depth guide looks into the realm of fertility-boosting smoothies, delving into the science behind the carefully selected components and their possible impact on reproductive health. We hope to give a tangible blueprint for couples facing similar issues by charting Sam and Sarah's actions. This road map, weaved with the threads of diet, lifestyle changes, and an unyielding spirit, carries the promise of guiding others toward the fulfillment of their parental ambitions.

The choice to share Sam and Sarah's story stems from the idea that knowledge empowers and that shared experiences can serve as a beacon of hope. Infertility is multidimensional, and the strategy for treating it should be as well. As we embark on this journey of fertility-boosting smoothies, we know that each couple's path to parenting is unique. However, the essential principles of nutrition and beneficial lifestyle choices are universally accepted.

Fertility issues are frequently linked to a slew of factors, ranging from genetic predispositions to environmental impacts. We address physical aspects while also contributing to the overall well-being of people and couples navigating this complex route by focusing on the synergy between nutrition and lifestyle changes.

The voyage ahead is divided into chapters, each of which provides insights into the important factors of fertility improvement. This book aims to empower couples with knowledge that goes beyond smoothie recipes, from understanding the underlying principles impacting fertility to investigating the significance of antioxidants and important nutrients.

We look into the broader landscape of lifestyle options in addition to the products and recipes. Exercise, stress management, and bad habits are examined to see how they affect reproductive health. Sam and Sarah's journey is more than simply the smoothies they added to their diet; it is a tribute to the holistic approach they took, recognizing that fertility is a reflection of total well-being.

In the sections that follow, we will look at specific smoothie recipes designed to boost fertility. These recipes are more than just a mash-up of ingredients; they are carefully curated blends meant to supply the critical nutrients required to sustain reproductive health. We welcome you to embark on this path with an open mind, ready to accept the possibility of fertility-boosting smoothies as an adjunct to your fertility enhancement plan.

As we negotiate the complexities of this book, we wish to not only provide you with information but also instil hope and resilience in you. Sam and Sarah's tale shines as a beacon, reminding us that the route to motherhood is fraught with difficulties, but it is also rich in opportunity for development, understanding, and unshakable perseverance. Let the journey to better fertility and health begins, one drink of a fertility-boosting smoothie at a time.

Overview of Fertility and Reproductive Health

Fertility, a fundamental aspect of human existence, entails the numerous processes that enable conception and the ability to bear new life. Beyond the ability to conceive, reproductive health involves the general well-being of the reproductive system within the context of an individual's health. A thorough understanding of fertility and reproductive health entails delving into the biological foundations, recognizing the multifactorial influences on fertility, understanding common fertility issues, and recognizing the psychological aspects associated with this deeply personal journey.

Biological Foundations

Fertility is a complicated interaction of biological processes within the human body. The combination of a sperm cell from the male and an egg cell from the female results in the development of a fertilized egg. This complicated dance takes place within the female reproductive system (ovaries, fallopian tubes, uterus, and cervix), as well as the male reproductive system (testes and related ducts). The menstrual cycle in females is crucial to fertility, a recurrent monthly process driven by hormonal variations that regulate ovulation—the release of an egg from the ovary.

Fertility Influencing Factors

Fertility is regulated by a variety of external and environmental factors in addition to biology. Fertility, a major determinant, peaks in the early twenties and then declines with age, especially dramatically in women. Fertility can also be affected by hormonal imbalances, structural abnormalities in reproductive organs, and hereditary factors.

Lifestyle decisions have a big impact on fertility. Nutrition, exercise, stress levels, and habits like smoking and drinking all play important factors in determining reproductive health. Environmental factors, such as exposure to poisons and pollution, add to the complication of reproductive results.

Common Fertility Issues

Many couples encounter infertility, which is defined as the inability to conceive after a year of regular, unprotected intercourse. It is critical to remember that infertility is not limited to women; male factors are responsible for roughly half of all infertility occurrences.

Common fertility difficulties encompass a wide range of disorders. Couples may face difficulties such as ovulatory disorders, structural abnormalities, sperm-related issues, and unexplained infertility. Endometriosis, polycystic ovarian syndrome (PCOS), and hormone imbalances can all have an impact on fertility in women, whereas male variables can include sperm production, motility, or structural abnormalities in the reproductive system.

The Psychological Aspect

Beyond the medical complications, reproductive issues frequently have a significant emotional and psychological impact. The emotional effect of infertility might be exacerbated by societal expectations and personal goals related to motherhood. Couples dealing with fertility challenges may suffer increased stress, anxiety, and feelings of inadequacy, highlighting the significance of a comprehensive approach to reproductive health that addresses both the medical and emotional elements.

The purpose of this overview is to present a concise yet comprehensive examination of fertility and reproductive health. The complex interaction of biological and environmental effects, as well as the complicated links between physical and emotional well-being, highlight the diverse nature of fertility. Individuals and couples can approach reproductive health with a nuanced understanding by appreciating these nuances, supporting informed decision-making and empowering themselves on their particular road to parenting.

Importance of Nutrition and Lifestyle in Fertility and Reproductive Health

Fertility and reproductive health are delicate dances of physiological systems that can be greatly altered by lifestyle and nutritional habits. Recognizing the significant influence of these elements is critical for people and couples looking to improve their odds of conception and promote general well-being.

Nutrition's Role in Reproductive Health

Nutrition is the foundation of reproductive health, providing the necessary building blocks for the complex processes of conception. A well-balanced, nutrient-dense diet is essential for the correct functioning of the reproductive system. Important vitamins and minerals, such as folate, zinc, and omega-3 fatty acids, play critical roles in fertility support. These nutrients help to regulate hormonal balance, promote egg and sperm health, and create a favorable environment for conception.

It is critical to consume a range of nutrient-dense foods, such as fruits, vegetables, whole grains, and lean proteins. These meals not only supply the necessary macronutrients and micronutrients but also fiber and antioxidants, which contribute to overall health and fertility.

Fertility and Antioxidants

Antioxidants, which are rich in fruits, vegetables, and nuts, protect against oxidative stress, which is a possible hazard to reproductive health. The reproductive system is especially prone to oxidative stress, which can impair both egg and sperm quality. Consuming antioxidant-rich meals reduces oxidative stress, creating an environment favorable to healthy reproductive cells and increasing fertility.

Maintaining a Healthy Weight

Weight control is an important component of reproductive health. Both being underweight and being overweight might interfere with hormonal balance and monthly regularity, impacting fertility. A healthy weight achieved and maintained by a balanced diet and regular exercise benefits overall reproductive function. This not only increases the odds of conception, but also leads to a healthy pregnancy.

Influence of Lifestyle on Hormonal Balance

Lifestyle decisions have a significant impact on hormonal balance, which is an important driver of reproductive health. Chronic stress, whether from work, relationships, or other sources, can disturb the delicate hormonal interaction, potentially impacting ovulation and sperm production. Stress management approaches, such as meditation, yoga, or mindfulness activities, might be beneficial in establishing hormonal balance.

Fertility and Physical Activity

Regular physical activity is an essential component of a healthy lifestyle, contributing not only to weight loss but also to overall well-being. Exercise improves blood circulation, increases hormonal balance, and reduces stress, all of which have a good impact on fertility. However, striking a balance is critical, as excessive exercise, particularly in women, can have a negative impact on reproductive health.

The Impact of Smoking and Alcohol

Unhealthy habits like smoking and excessive alcohol intake can have a major impact on fertility. Both chemicals have been related to lower sperm quality in men and can disturb female hormonal balance. Quitting smoking and limiting alcohol consumption are proactive efforts toward better reproductive health. These lifestyle modifications not only improve fertility but also add to both spouses' general health and set the foundation for a better pregnancy.

Environmental Factors

Environmental factors, such as exposure to certain chemicals and poisons, can have an impact on fertility. Being environmentally conscious, both at home and work, and limiting exposure to harmful reproductive toxins can all contribute to a healthier reproductive environment. This knowledge is especially important in today's society, as people are exposed to a wide range of environmental toxins regularly.

Importance of Hydration

Adequate hydration is sometimes disregarded, although it is essential for reproductive health. Water is needed for sustaining correct body functioning, such as cervical mucus formation, which is required for sperm travel. Staying hydrated benefits the reproductive system's general health and contributes to the optimal functioning of many physiological systems.

Collaboration with Healthcare Professionals

While lifestyle and nutrition can have a significant impact, it is critical to acknowledge the value of collaboration with healthcare specialists. Seeking the advice of reproductive specialists and healthcare providers can provide unique insights and solutions that are geared to individual needs. These professionals can perform extensive exams, identify particular concerns impacting fertility, and make tailored recommendations, such as dietary and lifestyle changes.

Nutrition and lifestyle choices are important parts of the complex tapestry that is reproductive health. A balanced lifestyle, nutrient-rich food, and making informed decisions all contribute to not only fertility but also overall well-being. Empowering people and couples with knowledge about these critical factors lays the groundwork for a proactive and holistic approach to reproductive health, supporting a journey to conception and motherhood that is rooted in optimal health and well-being.

CHAPTER TWO

UNDERSTANDING FERTILITY

Understanding fertility necessitates a careful examination of the elements that influence conception. Biological complexities, age, hormone balance, and genetic predispositions are all important factors. Common reproductive concerns, such as ovulatory disorders, structural abnormalities, and sperm-related issues, all contribute to the complex landscape of fertility challenges. Recognizing these characteristics enables individuals and couples to make informed decisions about their reproductive journey and, where necessary, seek focused interventions. Individuals can take proactive actions toward optimizing reproductive health and fulfilling the dream of parenthood by understanding the multifaceted nature of fertility.

Factors Affecting Fertility

Fertility, the ability to conceive and maintain a pregnancy, is the result of a complex interaction of biological, environmental, and lifestyle factors. Recognizing and grasping these components is critical for individuals and couples navigating the often perplexing journey to motherhood.

Age

Age is an important determinant of fertility. Fertility peaks in the early twenties and steadily declines with age, especially in women. Advanced maternal and paternal age are linked to an increased risk of infertility and pregnancy problems. Understanding the impact of age on fertility becomes critical for informed family planning decisions as people delay children for a variety of reasons.

Hormonal Balance

Hormones control the menstrual cycle, ovulation, and the creation of sperm. Imbalances, whether caused by polycystic ovarian syndrome (PCOS) or abnormalities in thyroid function, can have a substantial impact on fertility. Understanding hormonal health in depth is essential for resolving underlying disorders and optimizing reproductive potential.

Genetics

Genetic variables play a significant role in fertility results. Inherited diseases, chromosomal abnormalities, and family history can all have an impact on reproductive health. Couples with known hereditary issues may choose genetic counseling, which can provide insights into potential hazards and guide family planning decisions.

Reproductive Anatomy

For successful conception, the structural integrity of reproductive organs is critical. Endometriosis, uterine fibroids, and fallopian tube anomalies can all interfere with the normal process of egg fertilization and implantation. Addressing these structural issues frequently necessitates consultation with fertility professionals as well as tailored interventions.

Lifestyle Factors

Nutrition, exercise, and lifestyle choices all have an impact on reproductive health. A well-balanced diet rich in key nutrients promotes overall well-being, including specific vitamins and minerals important in fertility. Regular physical activity helps with not only weight loss but also hormonal balance. Smoking and excessive alcohol intake, on the other hand, hurt fertility and should be avoided for good reproductive health.

Environmental Exposures

Environmental variables, such as poisons, pollutants, and certain chemicals, can have an effect on fertility. Occupational dangers, lifestyle decisions, and geographical factors can all expose people to toxins that harm reproductive health. Awareness and actions to reduce exposure can help to create a more healthy reproductive environment.

Chronic Medical Conditions

Diabetes, autoimmune disorders, and certain infections can all have an impact on fertility. It is critical to manage these diseases in coordination with healthcare specialists to optimize reproductive health. Individuals with chronic health issues can approach family planning with a proactive and informed perspective thanks to careful monitoring and proper medical measures.

Medications and procedures

Certain medications and medical procedures, such as chemotherapy or radiation, may have fertility effects. Individuals having such procedures should have open discussions with their healthcare professionals to understand the potential consequences for reproductive health. In such circumstances, fertility preservation options may be investigated.

Psychological Stress

Long-term stress can have a significant impact on fertility. The stress response in the body can upset hormonal balance, potentially compromising ovulation and sperm quality. Stress management approaches, like as mindfulness, meditation, and relaxation practices, are critical for promoting overall reproductive health.

Weight and Body Composition

Both being underweight and being overweight can interfere with fertility. A healthy weight achieved and maintained by a balanced diet and regular exercise promotes hormonal balance and reproductive function. Lifestyle changes aimed at achieving a healthy weight benefit not only fertility but also overall health.

Understanding these multiple aspects equips individuals and couples on their fertility journey with a solid foundation. While some factors are out of one's control, proactive lifestyle choices and coordination with healthcare specialists can reduce risks and increase the chances of a healthy pregnancy and conception. Couples who are having difficulty conceiving are urged to seek tailored advice to address particular variables impacting their fertility, supporting a holistic approach to reproductive health.

Common Fertility Problems

The route to motherhood is not always easy, and many couples confront difficulties on the way to conception. Understanding typical reproductive concerns is critical for those traversing this difficult terrain since it enables them to seek proper help and remedies. Several variables that contribute to reproductive issues are discussed here:

Ovulatory Disorders

A major barrier to pregnancy is irregular or missing ovulation. Polycystic ovarian syndrome (PCOS) disrupts the normal ovulatory process, affecting egg release from the ovaries. It is critical to monitor menstrual cycles and identify anomalies to detect ovulatory problems.

Anatomical Imbalances in the Reproductive Organs

Anatomical anomalies within the reproductive organs can impair fertility. Uterine fibroids, polyps, or uterine shape anomalies can all interfere with the implantation of a fertilized egg. Diagnostic imaging and detailed examinations by fertility specialists aid in identifying and resolving structural issues.

Sperm-related Issues

Male factor infertility is a major contributor to reproductive problems. Fertility can be impacted by conditions that impair sperm production, motility, or morphology. Comprehensive sperm analysis and male reproductive health evaluations are required to identify potential sperm-related issues.

Unexplained Infertility

In some situations, couples may have fertility issues that have no obvious cause. Unexplained infertility can be emotionally draining because there may be no clear disease to target for treatment. Current research and breakthroughs in fertility diagnostics, on the other hand, may offer light on previously identified causes contributing to infertility.

Endometriosis is a disorder in which tissue comparable to the uterine lining grows outside the uterus. This can result in inflammation, scarring, and adhesion development, potentially affecting fertility. Endometriosis-related reproductive difficulties are frequently treated with laparoscopic surgery.

Hormonal Imbalances

Hormonal disruptions, whether caused by thyroid diseases or imbalances in reproductive hormones, can have an impact on fertility. Hormone tests and evaluations are critical for identifying and correcting hormonal abnormalities to enhance reproductive health.

Relative to age Female and male fertility both drop with age.

Women have a decrease in egg quantity and quality, while men may have a decrease in sperm quality. Advanced maternal and paternal age are linked to an increased risk of infertility and pregnancy problems.

Genetic Factors

Inherited genetic disorders or chromosomal abnormalities might lead to reproductive problems. Genetic testing and counseling may be advised, particularly for couples with known genetic issues.

Immunological Factors

Immunological Factors: Certain immune system reactions can hinder embryo implantation. Specialized assays can investigate the immunological mechanisms that contribute to recurrent pregnancy loss or implantation failure.

Lifestyle and Environmental Influences

Unhealthy lifestyle behaviors, such as smoking, excessive alcohol consumption, and poor diet, can all hurt fertility.

Toxin and pollutant exposure in the environment may potentially lead to reproductive difficulties. Lifestyle changes and limiting exposure to potentially dangerous components can be useful.

Navigating fertility challenges frequently necessitates coordination with fertility specialists, reproductive endocrinologists, and other healthcare providers. A thorough fertility examination is essential for identifying particular issues and adapting interventions to individual requirements. Adopting a holistic approach to parenting that covers both physical and mental components creates a resilient mindset on the road to motherhood. Couples dealing with fertility issues are advised to seek specialized counsel, with the understanding that each fertility journey is unique, and advances in reproductive medicine continue to give hope and possibilities.

CHAPTER THREE

BREAKING NUTRIENTS FOR FERTILITY

Navigating the complexity of fertility entails deconstructing the impact of numerous factors, such as age and hormone balance, as well as genetic predispositions and lifestyle decisions. The third chapter looks into the intricate interplay of these variables, shedding light on how dietary concerns are critical in promoting reproductive health. Understanding the importance of nutrients, including macro and micronutrients, reveals a strategy for sustaining the delicate balance essential for conception. This chapter establishes the framework for practical ideas that empower individuals and couples on their journey to better fertility and eventual pregnancy, covering everything from hydration necessities to fertility-boosting foods.

Essential Nutrients for Reproductive Health

Motherhood is a life-changing event that necessitates more than just eager anticipation—it necessitates a solid awareness of the nutritional fundamentals essential for optimal reproductive health. These vital nutrients perform a variety of roles in assisting the complex processes of conception and ensuring a healthy pregnancy. We delve into the relevance of each key nutrient in this comprehensive examination, shining light on their critical contributions to reproductive well-being.

Folate (Vitamin B9)

Folate is an essential nutrient for reproductive health, especially in the early stages of pregnancy. This water-soluble vitamin is required for the production and repair of DNA. Adequate folate levels are critical in developing embryos to prevent neural tube abnormalities. Folate is abundant in leafy greens like spinach and kale, lentils, and fortified cereals.

Beyond pregnancy preparation, folate is important in the pre-conception stage, regulating the health of both sperm and eggs. Individuals wanting to conceive should take folate supplements or eat a diet high in folate.

Iron

Iron, a vital iron, promotes reproductive health by increasing oxygen delivery throughout the body. A healthy blood supply is essential for the reproductive organs to operate properly. Iron-rich meals, such as red meat, chicken, fish, beans, and fortified cereals, help to avoid anemia and promote enough oxygen delivery to the reproductive system.

Iron deficiency can cause anemia, which can hurt fertility. Women of childbearing age should pay special attention to iron intake, ensuring that their nutritional needs are met to promote reproductive health.

Calcium

In addition to its well-known role in bone health, calcium is essential for uterine muscle function. A healthy pregnancy and successful conception require a fully functioning uterus. To maintain reproductive organ health, calcium-rich foods such as dairy products, leafy greens, and fortified plant-based milk should be included in the diet.

Calcium is essential not only for the uterus but also for the fetus's developing bones and teeth. The requirement for calcium increases during pregnancy, underscoring the continued necessity of this vitamin throughout the reproductive process.

Omega-3 Fatty Acids

Omega-3 fatty acids are essential for reproductive health, notably docosahexaenoic acid (DHA) and eicosapentaenoic acid (EPA). These fatty acids are necessary for the health of developing embryos because they contribute to the formation of the brain and central nervous system. Omega-3 fatty acids are abundant in fatty fish such as salmon and trout, as well as flaxseeds, chia seeds, and walnuts.

Omega-3 fatty acids are important because of their anti-inflammatory characteristics, which may improve fertility. Including these healthy fats in your diet is not only good for your reproductive health, but it is also good for your general health.

Zinc

Zinc, a trace element, is essential for reproductive health because it promotes DNA synthesis and sperm development. Adequate zinc levels have been linked to increased fertility in both men and women. Meat, dairy products, nuts, and seeds are dietary sources of zinc, making their inclusion in a well-balanced diet necessary for reproductive health.

Zinc is especially crucial in men for maintaining healthy sperm quality and quantity. Women benefit from zinc's role in cell division throughout early pregnancy as well.

Vitamin D

Also known as the "sunshine vitamin," vitamin D is essential for calcium absorption, bone health, and reproductive function. Vitamin D is mostly obtained from sunlight, fatty fish such as salmon and mackerel, egg yolks, and fortified dairy products.

In both men and women, vitamin D insufficiency has been related to infertility. It is critical to maintain enough levels of this vitamin for reproductive health and overall well-being.

Vitamin C

As a powerful antioxidant, vitamin C protects reproductive health. It protects reproductive cells from oxidative damage, which is critical for the quality of both eggs and sperm. Citrus fruits, berries, kiwi, and bell peppers are high in vitamin C and should be included in your diet.

Vitamin C's antioxidant capabilities extend to its involvement in preserving sperm from oxidative damage. Including vitamin C-rich foods in your diet helps to promote a healthy reproductive environment.

Vitamin E

Another antioxidant that protects cells from oxidative stress is vitamin E. Its role in reproductive cell protection helps to overall fertility. Vitamin E is abundant in nuts, seeds, vegetable oils, and green leafy vegetables.

Vitamin E is well-known for its function in overall cell health, and its antioxidant effects are especially advantageous to reproductive cells. Consuming a range of vitamin E-rich meals promotes fertility and reproductive health.

Protein

Protein is a macronutrient that is required for cell structure and function, including reproductive cells. Adequate protein consumption promotes general health by ensuring the availability of building blocks for reproductive tissues. Protein is found in lean meats, poultry, fish, dairy products, beans, and legumes.

Protein is an essential component of a well-balanced diet, helping to repair and develop tissues throughout the body. Protein promotes the formation of healthy eggs and sperm in the context of reproductive health.

Understanding the nuances of these critical nutrients allows for a more comprehensive approach to reproductive health. A healthy diet of these nutrients not only promotes fertility but also improves general health. Adopting a nutrient-rich diet becomes a foundational step as individuals and couples traverse the delicate path toward motherhood, feeding the body and creating an environment favorable to the awe-inspiring journey of conception and pregnancy.

Achieving optimal reproductive health necessitates a deliberate combination of lifestyle decisions, including nutrition. Individuals and couples can build an environment that maximizes the chance for a healthy conception and a successful pregnancy by recognizing the importance of these critical nutrients and incorporating them into daily dietary patterns. The path to motherhood begins with fueling the body, ensuring it has the essential nutrients required for the wonderful process of generating life.

Role of Antioxidants in Fertility

Beginning the journey to parenting is a life-changing experience, and understanding the nuanced role of antioxidants in conception becomes critical. The tremendous impact of antioxidants on reproductive health emerges as a cornerstone of preconception care as individuals and couples negotiate the path to conception. We look into the various ways antioxidants contribute to fertility, protecting both male and female reproductive systems and establishing the groundwork for a healthy pregnancy.

Defining Oxidative Stress

Overview of Oxidative Stress: Oxidative stress arises when the body's free radicals and antioxidants are out of equilibrium. Free radicals, which are highly reactive chemicals, can cause cellular damage by interfering with DNA, proteins, and lipids. This imbalance can cause oxidative damage, which has been related to a variety of health concerns, including fertility issues.

Impact of Oxidative Stress on Fertility

Cellular Damage: Reproductive cells, such as eggs and sperm, are especially vulnerable to oxidative stress. The integrity of genetic material can be compromised by oxidative stress, resulting in DNA fragmentation and decreased viability of these critical cells. In turn, this can have a detrimental influence on fertility and raise the chance of pregnancy problems.

Inflammation and Fertility: Oxidative stress contributes to chronic inflammation, which has been related to male and female infertility. Inflammation affects the delicate hormonal balance needed for optimal conception and can damage reproductive organ function.

The Antioxidant's Protective Role

Free Radical Neutralization: Antioxidants protect cellular health by neutralizing free radicals. Antioxidants protect cells from cellular harm by providing electrons to unstable free radicals. This protection is critical for the health and functionality of reproductive cells in the setting of fertility.

Antioxidants have an important function in preserving the integrity of cellular structures, particularly the membranes of eggs and sperm. This preservation is critical for ensuring that reproductive cells operate properly throughout fertilization and early embryo development.

Female Fertility and Antioxidants

Protecting Egg Quality: Female fertility is inextricably linked to egg quality. Oxidative stress can cause genetic mutations and chromosomal abnormalities to accumulate in eggs. Antioxidants help to preserve the integrity of eggs by reducing oxidative stress, increasing the odds of a successful conception.

Uterine Environment: The uterine environment is essential for early embryo development and implantation. Antioxidants may have a good effect on the uterine environment, making it more conducive to the implantation of a fertilized egg. This supportive environment is critical for the development of a healthy pregnancy.

Antioxidants and Male Fertility

Preserving Sperm Quality: Because of their high polyunsaturated fatty acid content, sperm are particularly sensitive to oxidative stress. Antioxidants play an important role in sperm quality preservation by avoiding oxidative damage to sperm DNA, preserving motility, and protecting against structural abnormalities. This preservation improves sperm functioning and raises the likelihood of successful conception.

Antioxidants Improve Sperm Function: Antioxidants improve the overall health and function of sperm.

Antioxidants support sperm viability by neutralizing free radicals, boosting their capacity to fertilize an egg. This improvement is critical for couples dealing with reproductive issues since good sperm function is a significant factor in successful conception.

Common Fertility Antioxidants

Vitamin C (Ascorbic Acid): This water-soluble vitamin is a powerful antioxidant with numerous advantages. Vitamin C protects both male and female reproductive cells from oxidative damage in the setting of fertility. Vitamin C is abundant in citrus fruits, strawberries, and bell peppers.

Tocopherol (Vitamin E) is a kind of vitamin E. Vitamin E, a fat-soluble antioxidant, protects cell membranes against oxidative damage. Its role in fertility is especially important since it contributes to the general health of reproductive cells. Vitamin E is found in abundance in nuts, seeds, and vegetable oils.

Selenium: This trace element is a component of antioxidant enzymes, such as glutathione peroxidase. Brazil nuts, seafood, and whole grains are all high in selenium.

Selenium aids antioxidant activity in protecting reproductive cells from oxidative damage.

Zinc: While zinc is well known for its function in reproductive health, it also has antioxidant effects. It helps antioxidant enzymes operate in both males and females. Meat, dairy products, nuts, and seeds are all good sources of zinc.

Coenzyme Q10 (CoQ10): CoQ10 is an antioxidant found in all cells that aid in energy production. Some research suggests that it has a good effect on egg and sperm quality. CoQ10 can be found in a variety of meals, including organ meats, fatty fish, and whole grains.

Dietary and Lifestyle Sources

A well-rounded, healthy diet is a core strategy to incorporate antioxidants into one's lifestyle. Antioxidant-rich foods include colorful fruits and vegetables, nuts, seeds, and whole grains. These foods' wide assortment of antioxidants provides comprehensive support for reproductive health.

Supplements: Supplements may be recommended in some circumstances to guarantee enough antioxidant intake. However, before introducing supplements into a fertility-focused program, it is critical to check with a healthcare expert. Individual requirements, as well as any conflicts with other medications or conditions, should be carefully examined.

Timing and Considerations

Prioritizing antioxidant-rich foods and leading a healthy lifestyle during the pre-conception phase establishes the framework for reproductive health. This proactive strategy guarantees that the body has the appropriate defenses in place to combat oxidative stress.

Antioxidant support is essential during pregnancy to enable continuing protection against oxidative stress and to support the developing fetus. Antioxidants have an impact that extends beyond conception, contributing to a healthy pregnancy and lowering the chance of problems.

Caution and Individualized Approaches

Individual Reactions: While antioxidants are useful, individual reactions may vary. What works for one individual may not work as well for another. To customize antioxidant solutions to individual needs, personalized techniques directed by healthcare professionals are required.

Balanced Approach: Excessive antioxidant use may not always result in increased fertility. A well-balanced approach to nutrition and supplementation is essential. Striking the appropriate balance ensures that the body receives the essential assistance while not tipping the scales too far in favor of excessive antioxidant activity.

The effect of antioxidants on fertility goes much beyond what is commonly understood about health. These protecting chemicals appear as key performers in the complex dance of conception and pregnancy. As individuals and couples embark on the path to motherhood, adopting an antioxidant-rich lifestyle becomes a proactive and powerful option. This option not only protects reproductive cells from oxidative stress, but also helps to create an environment suitable for the growth of new life.

The soothing benefits of antioxidants enhance the parenting journey, stressing the profound link between nutritional choices and the remarkable processes of conception and pregnancy.

CHAPTER FOUR

FERTILITY-BOOSTING SMOOTHIES

Elevate your fertility journey by introducing fertility-boosting smoothies into your daily routine. These nutrient-dense blends have been carefully crafted to naturally support reproductive health, offering both joy and sustenance to your journey to parenting. Begin by choosing items with fertility-boosting qualities, such as antioxidant-rich berries, fertility-friendly walnuts, and herbs such as maca. Create delectable combinations that match your taste preferences, providing a pleasurable way to focus your reproductive health. Remember to supplement your smoothie routine with a healthy lifestyle that includes regular exercise, stress management, and open communication with your healthcare provider. These smoothies are a delightful and healthy companion, feeding your body and spirit while you traverse the exciting road to parenthood, whether you're starting or enhancing your fertility journey.

Benefits of Smoothies for Fertility

Beginning the journey to motherhood is a life-changing event, and as individuals or couples travel this path, the importance of nutrition becomes increasingly important. Fertility-boosting smoothies, garnished with a vivid palette of nutrient-rich ingredients, emerge as more than just delectable beverages, but also as reproductive health allies. We dive into the numerous benefits that these nutritional combinations bring to the table, adding to the delicate processes of conception and fertility.

Comprehensive Nutrient Intake

Fertility-boosting smoothies provide a handy and effective approach to acquiring a wide range of vital nutrients in a single, tasty combination. These smoothies, which are high in vitamins, minerals, antioxidants, and other important substances, provide comprehensive sustenance that promotes overall reproductive health. The nutrient amalgamation guarantees that the body receives a varied spectrum of elements required for the delicate dance of conception.

Antioxidant Powerhouse

Oxidative Stress Defense: Fertility smoothies are high in antioxidants since they contain bright fruits like berries. These substances are critical in neutralizing free radicals, protecting reproductive cells from oxidative stress, and promoting a fertile environment. Smoothies help to maintain healthy eggs and sperm by reducing oxidative stress, which is essential for successful fertilization.

Hormonal Balance Support

Contribution of Vitamin B6: Bananas, a typical ingredient in fertility smoothies, include vitamin B6, a substance essential for hormonal balance. This vitamin helps with the synthesis and regulation of hormones that are essential for the menstrual cycle and overall reproductive health. Hormonal balance is critical for a regular and healthy reproductive cycle, which increases the likelihood of successful conception.

Folate for DNA Integrity

Leafy greens like spinach and kale, which are common in fertility smoothies, supply vital folate. This B vitamin is necessary for DNA synthesis and repair, as well as for proper cell division and the prevention of chromosomal abnormalities in reproductive cells. Folate's impact on cellular health extends to the early stages of embryonic development, underscoring its importance in the fertility landscape.

Omega-3 Fatty Acids for Reproductive Organs

Reproductive Organ Support: Flaxseeds and chia seeds add omega-3 fatty acids to fertility smoothies. These fats serve an important function in promoting the health of reproductive organs, hence promoting optimal conditions for conception. Omega-3 fatty acids have been related to better egg quality and sperm health, laying the groundwork for successful conception.

Protein for Cell Structure

Cellular Structure Support: Greek yogurt, a frequent protein source in fertility smoothies, contains critical amino acids that are required for cell development and repair. This includes reproductive cells' structural integrity, which supports their functionality and general health. Protein is essential for cell structure, including the building blocks of eggs and sperm.

Healthy Fats for Hormone Production

Avocados Help with Hormones: Creamy avocados, a delicious addition to fertility smoothies, provide healthful monounsaturated fats. These fats serve an important role in hormone production and aid in the absorption of fat-soluble vitamins, promoting a hormonal state favorable to reproduction. These nutritious fats benefit hormones like estrogen and progesterone, which are important for fertility.

Fiber for Gut Health

Balanced Gut Microbiome: Fiber-rich fruits, vegetables, and chia seeds are typically featured in fertility smoothies. This dietary component promotes a healthy gut flora, which improves overall health and may have an effect on fertility via the complex gut-brain axis. The gut microbiome is becoming more recognized as a role in reproductive health, and promoting its balance can have beneficial effects on fertility.

Adaptogenic Benefits

Potential of Maca Root: Some fertility smoothies include maca root, which is known for its adaptogenic capabilities. Maca may aid in stress adaptation, potentially boosting hormonal balance and general reproductive health. Adaptogens are acclaimed for their capacity to alter the body's response to stimuli, providing a holistic approach to aiding fertility's delicate hormonal dance.

Hydration and Detoxification

Hydration and cleansing: The liquid base of fertility smoothies, whether water or nut milk, aids with hydration, which is an important part of reproductive health. Proper hydration aids the body's natural detoxifying processes, hence promoting a healthy interior environment for conception. Hydration is essential for proper biological activities since it ensures that cells, particularly reproductive cells, operate in a fertile environment.

Weight Management

Supporting Healthy Body Weight: Because fertility is inextricably linked to body weight, weight management is critical for good reproductive function. Fertility smoothies, when consumed as part of a well-balanced diet, can help with weight control and overall health. Maintaining a healthy weight is linked to better fertility outcomes, and incorporating nutrient-dense smoothies fits with a holistic approach to overall well-being.

Convenience and Consistency

Fertility smoothies provide an easy and consistent way to incorporate fertility-supportive ingredients into your everyday routine. Smoothies allow flexibility in timing and smoothly integrate into everyday routines, whether eaten as a breakfast choice, snack, or post-workout refreshment. The ease of preparation and consumption encourages regular intake of fertility-supportive nutrients, emphasizing a long-term approach to reproductive health.

Psychological Benefits

Empowerment and Mindful Nutrition: Making and consuming fertility smoothies can have psychological benefits. Individuals feel empowered as they actively participate in their reproductive health journey. A mindful diet becomes a positive and intentional element of the reproductive process, connecting sustenance to the hopeful route to parenting.

Variety and Culinary Exploration

Flavors and textures vary: Fertility smoothies provide a large canvas for culinary play. The use of a variety of components provides for a wide range of flavors and textures, making the experience more enjoyable and minimizing nutritional monotony. Exploration of flavors and textures adds a joyful dimension to the fertility journey, turning nourishment into a sensual and enjoyable experience.

Personalization for Individual Needs

Individuals and Couples Can modify Recipes to particular Dietary tastes and Nutritional Needs. Fertility smoothies are highly adjustable, allowing people and couples to modify recipes to particular dietary tastes and nutritional needs. This customization guarantees that the smoothies meet the needs of each individual, providing a fully tailored approach to fertility treatment. Recognizing and responding to individual needs results in a tailored nutritional strategy that recognizes the individuality of each reproductive journey.

Fertility-boosting smoothies are a healthy and tasty addition to the route to parenting. Their advantages go beyond nutrition, embracing a variety of elements that influence reproductive health. Fertility smoothies become a delightful and empowering choice as individuals and couples negotiate the difficult route of conception—a testament to the fusion of science, flavor, and nourishing intention in the journey towards creating life. Fertility smoothies become a celebration of life and a nod to the complicated dance of nutrition and reproductive well-being with each drink.

Fertility-Boosting Smoothies' Key Ingredients

The skill of making fertility-boosting smoothies is a journey of deliberate nutrition, with each carefully selected ingredient playing a specific function in promoting reproductive health. As we begin this journey, let us look at the fundamental components that make up the foundation of these nutrient-rich elixirs, which contribute to the delicate processes of conception.

Berries: Antioxidant Powerhouses

Blueberries, strawberries, and raspberries are not only visually pleasing; they also contain a wealth of antioxidants. Berries contain chemicals that act as potent antioxidants, such as anthocyanins and vitamin C. These antioxidants are essential in countering oxidative stress, a process that can destroy reproductive cells. Individuals bring a blast of flavor as well as a robust defense against cellular damage by incorporating berries into fertility smoothies, producing an environment suitable for successful conception.

Leafy Greens: Folate and Essential Nutrients

Spinach, kale, and other leafy greens add a nutrient-dense punch to fertility-boosting smoothies. The most important of these is folate, a B vitamin that is required for DNA synthesis and cell division. Adequate folate intake is especially important during the first trimester of pregnancy to lower the incidence of neural tube abnormalities. Furthermore, leafy greens include a variety of nutrients, including iron and calcium, which contribute to general reproductive health. The addition of these nutrient-dense greens raises the nutritional profile of the smoothie, providing a foundation for cellular health and optimal fertility.

Bananas: Vitamin B6 for Hormonal Balance

Bananas add a touch of sweetness to fertility smoothies while also providing a good dose of vitamin B6. This vitamin aids in hormonal balance by regulating critical hormones involved in menstruation and reproductive health. Hormonal balance is essential for the regularity of menstrual cycles and ovulation, both of which have a substantial impact on fertility. Individuals contribute to the complicated dance of hormones by including bananas, establishing a pleasant environment for the goal of motherhood.

Avocado: Healthy Monounsaturated Fats

Avocados, which are creamy and rich, add more than just a delectable texture to fertility smoothies; they also add healthful monounsaturated fats to the mix. These lipids are essential for hormone synthesis and fat-soluble vitamin absorption. Avocados become a tasty ally in maintaining a reproductive-friendly hormonal environment because the body relies on several hormones for reproductive functions, including estrogen and progesterone. Avocados add to the overall pleasure of fertility-boosting smoothies, in addition to their nutritious benefits.

Greek Yogurt: Protein and Probiotics

With its thick and creamy consistency, Greek yogurt serves a dual purpose in fertility smoothies. It provides vital protein to the body, giving amino acids required for cellular construction and repair. Protein is an essential component of reproductive cells, ensuring their health and functionality. Furthermore, Greek yogurt contains probiotics, which promote healthy gut microbiota. According to emerging studies, there is a link between gut health and fertility, making probiotics a potentially beneficial part of fertility-boosting nutrition.

Flaxseeds and Chia Seeds: Omega-3 Fatty Acids

These tiny seeds are high in omega-3 fatty acids, which provide them a nutritional boost. Flaxseeds and chia seeds are high in alpha-linolenic acid, an omega-3 fatty acid with numerous health benefits. Omega-3 fatty acids are essential for the health of reproductive organs in the setting of fertility. According to research, omega-3 fatty acids may improve reproductive results, making these seeds valuable additions to fertility-boosting smoothies. Furthermore, their fiber content promotes digestive health, which improves general well-being.

Maca Root: Adaptogenic Properties

The ancient Peruvian superfood maca root adds adaptogenic characteristics to fertility smoothies. While there is limited scientific data on maca's direct impact on conception, traditional use and anecdotal reports suggest its potential to promote hormonal balance. As an adaptogen, maca may help the body adapt to stress, which is important for overall health and reproductive health. Its addition gives a distinct flavor character as well as adaptogenic assistance to the fertility-boosting concoction.

Water or Nut Milk: Hydration and Nutrient Transport

The liquid foundation of fertility smoothies, whether water, almond milk, or coconut water, has a purpose other than blending. It aids with hydration, which is an important part of reproductive health. Proper hydration aids in the body's natural detoxifying processes, resulting in a healthy interior environment for conception. Furthermore, the liquid foundation acts as a vehicle for the nutrients found in the other ingredients, boosting their absorption and use within the body.

Pineapple: Bromelain Enzyme

Pineapple adds a tropical flavor to fertility smoothies and contains bromelain, an enzyme with anti-inflammatory qualities. Although studies on bromelain's particular influence on fertility is scarce, several hypotheses suggest that it may aid in implantation. The pineapple's sweet and tart flavor adds a refreshing aspect to the smoothie, making it a welcome addition to the fertility-boosting arsenal.

Cinnamon: Blood Sugar Regulation

Cinnamon has potential benefits for blood sugar management in addition to its fragrant and warming properties. Because stable blood sugar levels are linked to better reproductive results, cinnamon is not only a tasty but also a practical ingredient. Cinnamon helps to create a balanced internal environment suitable to reproductive health by regulating blood sugar.

Walnuts: Omega-3 Fatty Acids and Antioxidants

With their distinct flavor and delicious crunch, walnuts provide a double advantage in fertility smoothies. They are high in omega-3 fatty acids, which enhance reproductive organ health and may increase fertility. Furthermore, walnuts provide antioxidants, reinforcing the smoothie against oxidative stress. Walnuts' combination of omega-3s and antioxidants makes them an important complement to the fertility-boosting diet.

Beets: Nitric Oxide Production

The earthy and colorful beetroot contributes nitrates to the fertility smoothie in addition to color. These nitrates can boost the generation of nitric oxide, a chemical involved in blood flow. While more research is needed to determine the direct influence on fertility, increased blood flow to reproductive organs is generally thought to be advantageous for reproductive health. The addition of beets to fertility-boosting smoothies provides a distinct depth to the nutrient profile.

The Final Blend: Crafting Fertility-Boosting Elixirs

The secret magic of fertility-boosting smoothies happens in the blender, not when the ingredients are combined. Making the ideal elixir requires a careful balance of flavors, textures, and nutrient-dense ingredients. Here's how to make a fertility-boosting smoothie step by step:

Choose a Base

Begin with a liquid base of your choice, such as water, almond milk, or coconut water. The base of the smoothie adds hydration and determines the overall texture.

Add Leafy Greens

Include a large handful of nutrient-dense leafy greens like spinach or kale. These greens serve as the smoothie's base, providing critical vitamins and minerals.

Introduce Berries

Combine berries high in antioxidants, such as blueberries, strawberries, or raspberries. These not only provide colorful tastes but also powerful antioxidants to the smoothie.

Creamy Texture with Avocado and Greek Yogurt

Half an avocado adds smoothness and healthy fats. Add a scoop of Greek yogurt for protein and probiotics, which will improve the texture as well as the nutritional value.

Omega-3 Boost with Seeds

To add omega-3 fatty acids, add a tablespoon each of flaxseeds and chia seeds. These seeds also provide fiber, which is beneficial to intestinal health.

Unique Flavors and Adaptogens

Try maca root powder for its distinct flavor and possibly adaptogenic effects. Begin with a small amount and gradually increase to your liking.

Additional Enhancements

Include pineapple slices for bromelain, cinnamon for flavor and possibly blood sugar management, and a handful of walnuts for omega-3s and texture.

Blend to Perfection

Blend all of the ingredients in a high-quality blender until smooth. If necessary, adjust the consistency by adding more liquid.

Garnish and Enjoy

Pour the smoothie into a glass and top with more berries, almonds, or cinnamon. Take time to enjoy the flavors and nurture both your body and your soul.

Personalize and Experiment

Feel free to experiment with different ingredients and proportions to make your fertility-boosting smoothie. Customize the recipe to your taste preferences and nutritional requirements.

Making fertility-boosting smoothies is more than just a culinary venture; it is a creative and conscious gesture to enhance reproductive health. Individuals and couples can enjoy a tasty and nourishing approach to fertility support by carefully selecting key components renowned for their fertility-enhancing characteristics and mixing them into a harmonic elixir. These nutrient-rich smoothies become a celebration of life with each drink, mixing science, flavor, and nourishing intention on the path to generating life.

CHAPTER FOUR

SMOOTHIE RECIPES

The introduction of nutrient-rich smoothie recipes reveals a delightful and purposeful path in the search for holistic well-being and fertility enhancement. These smoothies are more than just ingredient combinations; they are a harmonious marriage of science and flavor, painstakingly crafted to improve reproductive health. With each luscious sip, these concoctions contain a variety of antioxidants, vitamins, and minerals chosen for their fertility-promoting effects. Each recipe paints a canvas of flavors designed to feed the body on its journey toward conception, from the sumptuous combination of mixed berries in the Berry Bliss Fertility Smoothie to the exotic enticement of the Tropical Elixir Fertility Smoothie. These smoothies, infused with components known for their potential health benefits, not only tempt the tongue but also serve as delightful and nutritious partners in the complicated dance of producing life. Welcome to a world where every delectable sip is a celebration of health, flavor, and the pursuit of increased fertility.

Recipe 1: [Specific Fertility-Boosting Smoothie]

1. Berry Bliss Fertility Smoothie

Ingredients:

1 cup mixed berries (blueberries, strawberries, raspberries)

1 handful spinach

1 ripe banana

1/2 avocado

1/2 cup Greek yogurt

1 tablespoon flaxseeds

1 tablespoon chia seeds

1 cup almond milk

Ice cubes (optional)

Overview

Indulge in the delightful symphony of fertility-supporting ingredients with the Berry Bliss Fertility Smoothie. Bursting with antioxidants, vitamins, and minerals, this concoction is designed to nurture reproductive health.

Ingredient Highlights

Mixed Berries: Packed with antioxidants, these berries combat oxidative stress, creating an optimal environment for conception.

Spinach: A nutrient powerhouse, spinach provides essential vitamins and minerals, contributing to overall reproductive well-being.

Banana and Avocado: Rich in potassium and healthy fats, these fruits support hormonal balance, crucial for fertility.

Greek Yogurt: A protein and probiotic source, promoting reproductive cell health and a balanced gut microbiome.

Flaxseeds and Chia Seeds: Omega-3 fatty acids and fiber from these seeds enhance reproductive organ health and digestive well-being.

Almond Milk: The liquid base adds hydration and nutrients, facilitating the transport of fertility-supportive components.

Instructions

Place all ingredients in a blender.

Blend until smooth and creamy.

Adjust consistency with more almond milk if desired.

Pour into a glass, and relish the nutrient-rich goodness with each sip.

Customization Tips

Add a drizzle of honey for sweetness.

Include a scoop of protein powder for an extra boost.

Experiment with different greens like kale for variety.

Nourish your body with this Berry Bliss Fertility Smoothie, a flavorful and nutrient-packed ally on your fertility journey.

2. Tropical Paradise Fertility Smoothie

Ingredients

1 cup pineapple chunks

1/2 banana

1/2 cup mango chunks

1/2 avocado

1 tablespoon chia seeds

1 cup coconut water

Ice cubes (optional)

Ingredient Highlights

Pineapple: Rich in bromelain, an enzyme believed to support implantation.

Mango: Provides vitamin C and beta-carotene for reproductive health.

Chia Seeds: Omega-3 fatty acids for reproductive organ health.

Instructions

Blend all ingredients until smooth. Pour into a glass and enjoy the tropical goodness.

Customization Tip

For an extra citrus flavor, add a splash of lime juice.

3. Green Goddess Detox Fertility Smoothie

Ingredients

1 cucumber, peeled and sliced

1 green apple, cored and chopped

1 cup kale leaves

1/2 lemon, juiced

1 tablespoon spirulina powder

1 cup coconut water

Ice cubes (optional)

Ingredient Highlights:

Kale: Packed with folate and iron, supporting reproductive health.

Spirulina: Provides essential vitamins and minerals for detoxification.

Lemon Juice: Adds vitamin C, known for its antioxidant properties.

Instructions

In a blender, combine all of the ingredients and blend until smooth. Pour into a glass and relish the detoxifying green elixir.

Customization Tip

Include a handful of mint leaves for a refreshing twist.

4. Citrus Berry Burst Fertility Smoothie

Ingredients

1/2 cup blueberries

1/2 cup raspberries

1 orange, peeled and segmented

1/2 banana

1 tablespoon flaxseeds

1 cup almond milk

Ice cubes (optional)

Ingredient Highlights:

Blueberries and Raspberries: Packed with antioxidants for reproductive cell protection.

Flaxseeds: Omega-3 fatty acids for hormonal balance.

Instructions

Blend all ingredients until well combined. Pour into a glass and savor the refreshing citrus-berry fusion.

Customization Tip

Add a teaspoon of vanilla extract for a flavor boost.

5. Chocolate-Banana Bliss Fertility Smoothie

Ingredients

1 banana

2 tablespoons cacao powder

1 tablespoon almond butter

1/2 cup Greek yogurt

1 tablespoon hemp seeds

1 cup oat milk

Ice cubes (optional)

Ingredient Highlights:

Cacao Powder: Rich in antioxidants, promoting reproductive cell health.

Almond Butter: Provides healthy fats and vitamin E for fertility.

Instructions

Blend until creamy and smooth. Pour into a glass and treat yourself to a chocolate-infused fertility delight.

Customization Tip

Include a pinch of cinnamon for added warmth.

6. Pomegranate Powerhouse Fertility Smoothie

Ingredients

1 cup pomegranate seeds

1/2 cup strawberries

1/2 cup Greek yogurt

1 tablespoon pumpkin seeds

1 tablespoon honey

1 cup coconut water

Ice cubes (optional)

Ingredient Highlights:

Pomegranate Seeds: Loaded with antioxidants for reproductive health.

Pumpkin Seeds: Provide zinc, crucial for fertility.

Instructions

In a blender, combine all of the ingredients and blend until smooth. Pour into a glass and enjoy the antioxidant-rich power.

Customization Tip

Add a squeeze of lime juice for a zesty kick.

7. Vanilla Almond Joy Fertility Smoothie

Ingredients

1/2 cup almonds, soaked overnight

1/2 banana

1 tablespoon coconut flakes

1 teaspoon vanilla extract

1 tablespoon chia seeds

1 cup almond milk

Ice cubes (optional)

Ingredient Highlights:

Almonds: Provide vitamin E and healthy fats for reproductive health.

Coconut Flakes: Adds a tropical touch and medium-chain triglycerides.

Instructions

Blend until creamy. Pour into a glass and relish the nutty, vanilla-infused joy.

Customization Tip

Sprinkle a pinch of nutmeg for a festive flavor.

8. Raspberry Lemonade Fertility Smoothie

Ingredients

1 cup raspberries

1 lemon, juiced

1/2 banana

1 tablespoon flaxseeds

1 tablespoon honey

1 cup coconut water

Ice cubes (optional)

Ingredient Highlights:

Raspberries: Packed with antioxidants and vitamin C.

Flaxseeds: Omega-3 fatty acids for hormonal support.

Instructions

Blend until smooth. Pour into a glass and enjoy the zesty and sweet raspberry lemonade fusion.

Customization Tip

Garnish with a lemon slice for a decorative touch.

9. Mango Turmeric Wellness Fertility Smoothie

Ingredients

1 cup mango chunks

1/2 teaspoon turmeric powder

1 tablespoon ginger, grated

1/2 avocado

1 tablespoon hemp seeds

1 cup coconut water

Ice cubes (optional)

Ingredient Highlights:

Turmeric: Anti-inflammatory properties for reproductive wellness.

Ginger: Supports digestion and adds a zing to the smoothie.

Instructions

Blend until well combined. Pour into a glass and savor the tropical and anti-inflammatory wellness blend.

Customization Tip

Sprinkle a pinch of black pepper to enhance turmeric absorption.

10. Cinnamon Apple Pie Fertility Smoothie

Ingredients

1 apple, cored and chopped

1/2 banana

1/2 teaspoon cinnamon

1 tablespoon almond butter

1 cup oat milk

Ice cubes (optional)

Ingredient Highlights

Cinnamon: Supports blood sugar regulation for reproductive health.

Almond Butter: Adds creaminess and vitamin E.

Instructions

Blend until creamy and aromatic. Pour into a glass and enjoy the comforting taste of cinnamon apple pie.

Customization Tip

Top with a sprinkle of granola for added texture.

11. Kiwi Basil Bliss Fertility Smoothie

Ingredients

2 kiwis, peeled and sliced

1/2 cup basil leaves

1/2 banana

1 tablespoon chia seeds

1 tablespoon honey

1 cup coconut water

Ice cubes (optional)

Ingredient Highlights

Kiwi: High in vitamin C and antioxidants for reproductive health.

Basil: Adds a unique flavor and potential anti-inflammatory benefits.

Instructions

Blend until smooth. Pour into a glass and relish the unique and refreshing kiwi basil fusion.

Customization Tip

Add a handful of spinach for a nutritious boost.

Feel free to experiment with these recipes, adjusting ingredients to suit your taste and nutritional preferences. Enjoy the delightful and nutrient-packed journey toward enhanced fertility!

Recipe 2: Citrus Mint Revitalizer Fertility Smoothie

Ingredients

1 cup mixed citrus (orange, grapefruit segments)

1/2 cup strawberries

1/2 banana

1/2 cucumber, peeled and sliced

1 tablespoon fresh mint leaves

1 tablespoon chia seeds

1 cup coconut water

Ice cubes (optional)

Ingredient Highlights:

Citrus Fruits: Rich in vitamin C and antioxidants, promoting reproductive cell health.

Mint Leaves: Adds a refreshing flavor and potential digestive benefits.

Cucumber: Hydrating and contains silica, crucial for connective tissue health.

Instructions

Blend all ingredients until smooth. Pour into a glass and relish the citrusy mint revitalization.

Customization Tip

Include a small knob of ginger for an added zing.

Overview

Dive into a refreshing oasis of fertility support with the Citrus Mint Revitalizer. This vibrant smoothie brings together a medley of citrus fruits, strawberries, and the invigorating touch of mint. Loaded with fertility-enhancing nutrients, this concoction not only tantalizes the taste buds but also provides a burst of vitality to support your reproductive wellness journey.

Recipe 3: Blueberry Kale Powerhouse Fertility Smoothie

Ingredients

1 cup blueberries

1 cup kale leaves

1/2 banana

1/2 cup Greek yogurt

1 tablespoon almond butter

1 tablespoon hemp seeds

1 cup almond milk

Ice cubes (optional)

Ingredient Highlights:

Blueberries: Antioxidant-rich, supporting reproductive cell protection.

Kale: A nutrient-dense green, providing essential vitamins and minerals.

Almond Butter and Hemp Seeds: Offer healthy fats and protein for hormonal balance.

Instructions

Blend until creamy. Pour into a glass and indulge in the nutrient-packed goodness of the Blueberry Kale Powerhouse.

Customization Tip

For a bit of sweetness, add a spoonful of honey.

Overview

Elevate your fertility journey with the Blueberry Kale Powerhouse. This nutrient-dense smoothie combines the antioxidant power of blueberries with the nutritional richness of kale, creating a delicious blend that nourishes your body from within. Packed with vitamins, minerals, and essential nutrients, this smoothie is a vibrant addition to your fertility-boosting repertoire.

Feel free to experiment with these recipes, adjusting ingredients based on your preferences and nutritional needs. Enjoy the diverse and delicious world of fertility-boosting smoothies

CHAPTER SIX

REPRODUCTIVE HEALTH AND LIFESTYLE

The delicate tango between lifestyle choices and reproductive health is a critical component of the road to pregnancy. A holistic approach to well-being goes beyond fertility-focused interventions to include a range of lifestyle factors that all contribute to reproductive vitality. Understanding and appreciating these aspects empowers individuals and couples on their journey to naturally nurture fertility.

Nutrition: The Basis of Reproductive Wellness

A well-balanced, nutrient-dense diet is the foundation for reproductive health. Essential nutrients like folate, iron, omega-3 fatty acids, and antioxidants are critical for hormonal balance, reproductive organ function, and reproductive cell protection.

Hydration: Adequate water intake is essential for hormone regulation, nutrition transport, and the overall health of reproductive organs. Staying hydrated creates ideal conditions for conception.

Weight Control: Reproductive health must maintain a healthy weight. Both being underweight and being overweight can alter hormonal balance, affecting menstrual cycles and fertility. A healthy diet and frequent exercise are essential for striking a balance.

Physical Activity Boosts Fertility

Regular Exercise:=

Physical activity helps to maintain hormonal balance, regulate menstrual cycles, and improve blood supply to reproductive organs. Moderate exercise helps with weight management and reduces stress, creating an ideal environment for conception.

Mind-Body Practices: Including mind-body practices like yoga and meditation not only reduces stress but also improves relaxation and emotional well-being. Chronic stress can negatively alter reproductive hormones, thus stress management is critical.

Restorative Pose: Sleep Hygiene

Quality Sleep

Adequate and high-quality sleep is critical for the control of reproductive hormones and overall health. Sleep disruptions can disrupt hormonal balance, influencing menstrual cycles and fertility.

Circadian Rhythms: Adhering to natural circadian rhythms promotes hormone production. Consistent sleep-wake cycles and exposure to natural light during the day help to regulate hormones such as melatonin and cortisol, which aid in reproductive health.

Stress Management: Bridging the Mind-Body Gap

Techniques for Mindfulness and Relaxation

Stress has a deleterious impact on reproductive health by affecting hormone levels. Mindfulness, deep breathing, and other relaxation practices reduce stress, resulting in a fertile atmosphere.

Holistic Approaches: Exploring holistic approaches like acupuncture and massage therapy may aid in reducing stress and promoting overall well-being. These approaches deal with both the physical and emotional elements of reproduction.

Environmental Factors: Making a Fertility-Friendly Environment

Toxin Avoidance

It is critical to limit exposure to environmental toxins such as certain chemicals and pollutants. These chemicals have the potential to alter hormonal balance and impair reproductive function.

Adopting fertility-friendly habits, such as avoiding excessive alcohol use and quitting smoking, has a positive impact on reproductive health. These lifestyle changes help to create a more favorable interior environment for conception.

Monitoring Reproductive Health: Making Informed Decisions Menstrual Cycle Tracking:

Menstrual cycle awareness provides vital insights into reproductive health. Regular tracking aids in the detection of probable anomalies as well as favorable fertility windows for conception.

Regular medical check-ups with healthcare experts enable the discovery and control of any underlying reproductive health disorders. Early intervention has been shown to increase reproductive results.

Each choice in the complicated interplay between lifestyle and reproductive health contributes to the individual's or couple's total well-being. Individuals can empower themselves on the path to better fertility by adopting a holistic approach that includes nutrition, physical exercise, stress management, and environmental concerns. Adopting a reproductive health-promoting lifestyle not only aids in conception but also creates the groundwork for a healthy and balanced existence.

Impact of Diet on Fertility

The relationship between nutrition and fertility is an important part of reproductive health since what we eat has a substantial impact on hormonal balance, reproductive organ function, and overall well-being. Adopting a fertility-friendly diet is about establishing an environment within the body that effectively supports the numerous processes that lead to pregnancy. Here's an in-depth look at how nutrition affects fertility:

Nutrients Required for Reproductive Health

Folate (B-vitamin) is necessary for the development of a healthy embryo since it is required for DNA synthesis and cell division. It also aids in the prevention of neural tube abnormalities during the early stages of pregnancy.

Iron: Adequate iron levels are required to prevent anemia, promote healthy ovulation, and sustain the increased blood volume during pregnancy.

Omega-3 Fatty Acids: Found in fatty fish, flaxseeds, and walnuts, omega-3 fatty acids help to balance hormones, reduce inflammation, and aid in the development of the embryonic brain and eyes.

Antioxidants: Antioxidants such as vitamins C and E, as well as selenium and zinc, protect reproductive cells from oxidative stress and improve overall fertility.

Hormonal Balance and Blood Sugar Regulation Complex Carbohydrates: Choosing whole grains over refined carbohydrates helps regulate blood sugar levels, preventing insulin spikes that can disrupt hormonal balance and ovulation.

Healthy Fats: Consuming healthy fats such as avocados, almonds, and olive oil promotes hormone production. Hormone balance is essential for menstrual regularity and fertility.

Weight Management and Fertility

Body Mass Index (BMI): A healthy weight is essential for fertility. Ovulation and menstrual cycles can be disrupted by both underweight and overweight circumstances. A nutritious diet and a healthy weight promote reproductive health.

Protein Intake

Getting enough protein from foods such as lean meat, poultry, fish, lentils, and dairy helps muscular development and offers critical amino acids for reproductive tissues.

Hydration and Caffeine Intake

Water Consumption

Staying hydrated is important for overall health and helps the cervical mucus, which aids in sperm motility. Dehydration can cause mucus to thicken, impeding sperm motility.

Caffeine Moderation: While moderate caffeine usage is generally seen as healthy, high consumption has been associated with fertility difficulties. Choosing herbal teas and reducing caffeinated beverages can help with reproductive health.

Fertility and Plant-Based Diets

Vegan and vegetarian diets

Vegetarian and vegan diets that are well-planned can include all of the nutrients required for fertility. It is critical to pay attention to vital minerals such as iron, vitamin B12, and omega-3 fatty acids.

Plant-Based Proteins: Including plant-based protein sources such as beans, tofu, and quinoa in your diet offers an appropriate intake of key amino acids that are important for reproductive health.

Trans Fat Avoidance Dietary Factors: A high consumption of trans fats, which are commonly present in processed and fried foods, has been linked to an increased risk of ovulatory infertility.

Excess Sugar: Diets heavy in added sugars can cause insulin resistance, which can interfere with ovulatory activity. Choosing whole, unprocessed foods helps to keep blood sugar levels constant.

Processed Meats: Limiting your consumption of processed meats is recommended because some studies have linked them to lower fertility. It is healthier to use lean protein sources.

Fertility-Boosting Nutrients in Specific Foods

Walnuts:

Walnuts, which are high in omega-3 fatty acids and antioxidants, promote reproductive health and may boost sperm quality.

Berries: High in antioxidants, berries protect reproductive cells from oxidative stress and increase fertility.

Spinach, kale, and other leafy greens are high in folate, iron, and other elements important for reproductive health.

Fatty fish, such as salmon, mackerel, and sardines, provide omega-3 fatty acids, which promote hormonal balance and fertility.

Adopting a fertility-conscious diet is a proactive step in creating a fertile environment. A well-balanced, whole-foods-based diet guarantees adequate nutritional intake, hormonal balance, and weight maintenance. While dietary variables are important, they are only one element of holistic fertility treatment. A balanced diet combined with a healthy lifestyle, frequent exercise, and stress management constitutes a complete strategy for promoting reproductive well-being. Consultation with a healthcare expert or a nutritionist can provide tailored advice based on individual needs, ultimately fostering the route to a healthy and successful pregnancy.

Exercise and Fertility

The interaction between exercise and fertility is a complex one, involving both physiological and psychological aspects. Regular physical activity has been linked to a variety of health advantages, including increased cardiovascular function, weight management, and improved mental well-being. However, the effect of exercise on fertility is complex, and striking the appropriate balance is critical. Here's a thorough examination of the relationship between exercise and fertility:

The Benefits of Regular Exercise Weight Management

A healthy weight is essential for reproductive health. Regular exercise aids in the attainment and maintenance of a healthy weight, lowering the risk of fertility concerns linked with both underweight and overweight situations.

Hormonal Balance: Exercise has a good effect on hormonal balance, including insulin sensitivity and sex hormone regulation. This equilibrium is required for normal menstrual cycles and proper reproductive function.

Blood Circulation

Physical exercise promotes blood circulation, ensuring that reproductive organs receive an adequate supply of oxygen and nutrients. Improved blood flow can help with fertility.

Stress Reduction: Exercise is an effective stress reliever, and stress management is critical for reproductive health. High amounts of stress can disturb hormonal balance and menstrual cycles, thus impacting fertility.

Finding the Right Balance

Moderation is Key

While regular exercise is healthy, excessive or hard workouts may be detrimental to fertility. High-intensity training can cause menstrual cycle disturbances, especially in women with minimal body fat.

Avoiding Extreme Conditions: Participating in extreme endurance exercises or sports can occasionally result in amenorrhea (absence of menstruation), which can have an impact on fertility. It is critical to strike a balance and avoid extremes.

Individual Variability: The effect of exercise on fertility varies from person to person. Genetics, overall health, and individual stress reactions all play a part in how exercise affects reproductive function.

Types of Exercise and Fertility

Cardiovascular Exercise

Moderate-intensity cardiovascular exercise, such as brisk walking, cycling, or swimming, is usually thought to improve fertility. It boosts general health, aids in weight loss, and promotes blood circulation.

Strength Training: Including strength training activities in your routine helps you build and maintain muscular mass, which contributes to your overall fitness. It also helps with weight loss and hormonal balance.

Yoga and Mind-Body activities: Mind-body activities such as yoga and meditation not only provide physical advantages, but they also help with stress reduction and mental well-being, which influences fertility positively.

Timing of Exercise in the Menstrual Cycle

Follicular Phase: The follicular phase, which begins when menstruation begins, is often a good time for more strenuous workouts. During this phase, hormonal changes may improve workout performance.

Luteal Phase

Some women may prefer lower-intensity activities during the luteal phase, which occurs after ovulation. This phase is closer to menstruation and may be related to energy fluctuations.

Exercise and Male Fertility

While the effects of exercise on male fertility have received less attention than that of female fertility, some evidence suggests that moderate exercise may have a good effect on semen quality.

Avoiding Overheating

Excessive heat-generating activities, such as regular hot tub use or lengthy riding, may influence sperm production.

Moderate activity and avoiding harsh circumstances are recommended.

When to Seek Professional Guidance

Individuals with prior reproductive difficulties or medical disorders should seek the advice of a healthcare expert before making significant modifications to their workout regimens.

Fertility Treatments: Medical supervision is essential for those receiving fertility treatments. Exercise suggestions may be modified depending on the treatment strategy.

The association between exercise and fertility is dynamic, impacted by a variety of factors that are unique to each person. By including modest and enjoyable physical activity into one's routine, one can contribute to overall reproductive well-being. Listening to one's body, paying attention to menstrual cycles, and getting professional help when necessary are all important parts of negotiating the complicated interplay between exercise and fertility. Finally, a comprehensive approach that incorporates a healthy lifestyle, nutritious food, and mindful exercise prepares the body for optimal reproductive health and the path toward conception.

Stress Management for Improved Reproductive Health

Reproductive health is inextricably intertwined with overall well-being, and stress can have a major impact on reproductive results. Stress, whether chronic or acute, can influence hormonal balance, disrupt menstrual cycles, and impair fertility in both men and women. As a result, employing appropriate stress management measures is critical for achieving optimal reproductive health.

Understanding the Stress-Reproductive Health Connection

Stress causes the release of cortisol and other stress hormones, which can disrupt the delicate balance of reproductive hormones including estrogen and progesterone. Stress-related hormonal imbalances in women can cause irregular menstrual periods, and ovulatory dysfunction, and even impair the effectiveness of assisted reproductive technologies such as in vitro fertilization (IVF). Stress in men can impair sperm production, motility, and overall sperm quality.

Effects of Chronic Stress on Fertility

Chronic stress can cause a permanent state of heightened arousal in the body, resulting in consistently increased cortisol levels. This can affect the normal operation of the hypothalamus and pituitary glands, which regulate reproductive hormones. Chronic stress in women can lead to polycystic ovarian syndrome (PCOS) or amenorrhea, but in men, it can cause erectile dysfunction and diminished sperm production.

Effective Stress Management Techniques

Mindfulness Meditation: Deep breathing exercises and meditation are examples of mindfulness activities that can assist in managing the stress response. Incorporating these approaches throughout daily life will help you relax and lessen the physiological effects of stress on reproductive function.

Regular Exercise: Studies have shown that physical activity lowers stress hormones and improves mood.

Regular, moderate exercise not only improves general health but also helps to manage stress and its possible impact on reproductive health.

Balanced Nutrition: Maintaining hormonal balance requires a well-balanced, nutrient-rich diet. Certain nutrients, including omega-3 fatty acids and antioxidants, have been associated with increased fertility and stress resilience.

Adequate Sleep: Quality sleep is essential for general health and helps with stress management. Healthy sleep habits can improve reproductive hormones and promote optimal fertility.

Social Support: Creating a strong support system can help people cope with stress. Sharing worries and seeking support from friends, family, or support groups can help ease the emotional load that comes with fertility issues.

Professional Guidance and Counseling

Individuals who are suffering substantial stress due to fertility difficulties may benefit from getting professional help from reproductive health counselors or therapists.

Professional help can offer coping strategies, emotional support, and a safe space to negotiate the complicated emotions that come with fertility issues.

Recognizing the complex relationship between stress and reproductive health is the first step toward effective management. Implementing a comprehensive approach that considers physical, emotional, and psychological well-being can help enhance reproductive outcomes. Individuals and couples can improve their reproductive health by adopting stress management practices into their daily lives, increasing their chances of successful conception and a healthy pregnancy.

CHAPTER SEVEN

HABITS TO AVOID

The process that leads to conception entails more than just timing and patience; it necessitates a deliberate approach to lifestyle choices. Individuals and couples seeking optimal reproductive health must avoid certain practices. From abstaining from smoke and excessive drinking to managing stress and eating a well-balanced diet, these habits are critical in creating an environment suitable for healthy conception. This inquiry delves into bad behaviors to avoid, arming those on the path to motherhood with the knowledge they need to promote fertility and lay the groundwork for a healthy and enjoyable pregnancy.

Harmful Habits and Their Impact on Reproductive Health

Understanding the effects of hazardous habits on reproductive health is critical for people and couples attempting to conceive. Unhealthy lifestyle choices can have an impact on fertility, affecting both male and female reproductive systems. In this detailed investigation, we deconstruct the impact of specific habits on reproductive well-being and emphasize the necessity of avoiding actions that may impede the path to parenthood.

Smoking and Tobacco Use Impact on Reproductive Health

Women: Smoking can interfere with hormone production, lower egg quality, and increase the risk of miscarriage.

Smoking has been associated with poorer sperm quality, lower sperm count, and erectile dysfunction in men.

Long-Term Consequences

Fertility treatments are more likely to be unsuccessful.

Pregnancy problems, such as preterm birth and low birth weight, are increased.

Excessive Alcohol Consumption Impact on Reproductive Health

Women: Excessive alcohol use can alter menstrual cycles, impede ovulation, and contribute to fertility problems.

Alcohol can reduce sperm production and motility in men.

Considerations for Preconception

During the preconception phase, both partners should limit their alcohol consumption.

Chronic alcohol usage may impair fertility in the long run.

Illicit Drug Use Impact on Reproductive Health

In both men and women, illicit drugs can disturb hormonal balance and impede reproductive functions.

The usage of drugs may jeopardize the success of reproductive therapies.

Recovery and Fertility

Seeking therapy for and recovering from substance use disorders is critical to regaining reproductive health.

Drug use can have long-term implications on fertility.

Poor Nutrition and Diet Impact on Reproductive Health

An inadequate diet can result in a lack of vital nutrients required for reproductive function.

A poor diet might cause irregular menstrual periods and lower sperm quality.

Fertility Enhancement Techniques

Adopting a balanced diet rich in vitamins, minerals, and antioxidants supports reproductive health.

In cases of recognized deficits, nutrient supplementation may be advised.

Overexertion and Extreme Exercise Impact on Reproductive Health

Women's menstrual cycles can be disrupted by intense or excessive exercise, resulting in irregular ovulation.

Men's sperm quality may suffer as a result of overtraining.

Approach with Balance

Physical activity that is moderate and pleasurable promotes reproductive health.

Women who are attempting to conceive might consider timing their exercise with their menstrual cycle.

Overheating and Sauna Use Impact on Reproductive Health

Men's sperm production and motility can be temporarily affected by prolonged exposure to high temperatures.

Elevated temperatures may have an effect on egg quality in women.

Preconception Precautions:

Heat exposure, especially saunas and hot baths, should be avoided throughout the preconception period.

Maintaining a temperature equilibrium promotes reproductive health.

Chronic Stress and Poor Stress Management Impact on Reproductive Health

Chronic stress can throw off hormonal balance, resulting in irregular menstrual cycles and fertility issues.

Men's sperm quality may be affected by stress.

Stress Reduction on a Holistic Level

Stress-reduction practices such as mindfulness and relaxation improve reproductive health.

Seeking mental health help can help with general stress management.

Lack of Regular Health Check-ups Impact on Reproductive Health

Neglecting regular health check-ups may result in undiscovered fertility concerns.

Untreated health issues can lead to long-term reproductive difficulties.

Preconception Assessments

Before trying conception, both spouses should have regular health check-ups to identify and address any potential health issues.

Early intervention improves fertility outcomes.

Recognizing the impact of bad habits on reproductive health is the first step toward a fertility-friendly lifestyle.

Avoiding these harmful activities and using preventive measures such as a balanced diet, moderate exercise, and stress management pave the way for excellent reproductive health. Adopting a holistic approach to health benefits not only successful conception but also the establishment of a foundation for a healthy and enjoyable pregnancy experience.

Factors Influencing Fertility in the Environment

Environmental influences weave a substantial and sometimes unnoticed story in the intricate fabric of factors influencing fertility. The modern world exposes people to a plethora of drugs, toxins, and lifestyle variables that may have an impact on reproductive health. This in-depth investigation tries to understand the intricacies of environmental influences influencing fertility, giving insight on the various causes and potential repercussions for both men and women.

Endocrine Disruptors: The Hormonal Culprits Sources

Plasticizers (Bisphenol A, Phthalates): These chemicals are found in plastics, food packaging, and personal care items.

Pesticides and herbicides: Pesticides and herbicides are found in conventionally grown produce and agricultural techniques.

Industrial Chemicals: Endocrine disruptive substances are released throughout certain production processes.

Influence on Fertility

Women: Endocrine disruptors can alter menstrual cycle, ovulation, and hormonal balance.

Men: Sperm quality and reproductive hormone levels can be compromised, potentially resulting in infertility.

Air Pollution: Breathing in Reproductive Risks

Airborne Threats

Particulate Matter (PM): Particulate Matter (PM) is emitted by vehicle exhaust, industrial activity, and combustion processes.

Nitrogen Dioxide (NO2) and Sulphur Dioxide (SO2): Both are common in urban areas.

Volatile Organic Compounds (VOCs): Released from household products and industrial sources.

Reproductive Consequences

Women and Men: Long-term exposure to air pollution has been linked to decreased fertility, an increased chance of miscarriage, and poor pregnancy outcomes.

Fetuses in Development: Air pollution has been connected to developmental problems in fetuses.

Heavy Metals: The Weight of Reproductive Toxicity Common Heavy Metals

Lead: Present in old pipes, paint, and certain occupational settings.

Mercury: Mercury pollutes some fish and seafood.

Cadmium: Cadmium is a heavy metal found in fertilizers, tobacco smoke, and industrial operations.

Reproductive Implications

Heavy metals can have an effect on sperm quality, motility, and DNA integrity in men.

Women: Pregnancy exposure may contribute to developmental difficulties in the fetus.

Lifestyle Choices and Reproductive Health

Secondhand smoke and smoking

Impact on Women: Smoking has been associated to decreased ovarian reserve, an increased chance of miscarriage, and early menopause in women.

Impact on Men: Smoking can reduce sperm quality and contribute to erectile dysfunction in men.

Alcohol and Drug Use

Excessive alcohol consumption and illegal drug use can disturb hormonal balance and lead to reproductive issues in both men and women.

Occupational Exposures: Workplace Dangers

Occupational Risks

Certain vocations need exposure to chemicals, radiation, or extreme heat.

Agricultural laborers, industrial workers, and healthcare professionals may be exposed to reproductive risks.

Safety precautions

Risks can be reduced by following safety requirements, wearing protective equipment, and sharing concerns with employers.

Evaluation and adaptation to potential occupational dangers may be part of preconception planning.

Lifestyle Habits and Dietary Choices

Dietary Exposures

Pesticides are consumed through conventionally grown produce.

Contaminants are consumed through high-mercury-content fish and seafood.

Mitigation Strategies

Choosing organic products and limiting your consumption of high-mercury fish.

Including a variety of nutrient-rich foods that promote reproductive health in one's diet.

Preconception Planning and Environmental Awareness

Preconception Period:

During the preconception period, it is critical to be aware of environmental exposures.

To enhance reproductive health, both spouses should make educated decisions.

Detoxification Considerations

Some people may look into detoxification programs in order to decrease their exposure to environmental toxins.

Such methods should be approached with caution and professional advice.

Understanding the complex interaction between environmental influences and fertility is critical for individuals considering motherhood. While total avoidance of environmental exposures may be impracticable, informed decision-making and lifestyle changes can make a major difference in reproductive health. Individuals and couples can negotiate the difficult terrain of environmental influences with knowledge and proactive measures, producing an atmosphere conducive to successful conception and a good pregnant journey.

CHAPTER EIGHT

MEDICAL CONSULTATION AND ASSISTANCE

The importance of medical consultation and assistance in the quest for motherhood cannot be emphasized. Collaboration with healthcare specialists becomes an essential component, providing specialized insights and assistance customized to specific circumstances. Fertility specialists undertake comprehensive exams, examining hormone profiles, reproductive anatomy, and lifestyle variables to develop tailored programs. When appropriate, this collaborative approach extends to investigating assisted reproductive technologies such as in vitro fertilization (IVF) or fertility drugs.

Medical assistance, on the other hand, goes beyond diagnostics, delving into the emotional aspects of the reproductive process. Mental health specialists provide vital assistance in navigating the emotional complications associated with reproductive challenges for individuals and couples. In inclusive medical consultations, open talks, inquiries, and active participation in decision-making are not only encouraged but also required. This comprehensive approach ensures that the path to conception is not only medically competent but also emotionally helpful, giving people the resources and advice required for a successful reproductive journey.

Knowing When to Seek Professional Advice on Fertility Matters

The path to parenthood is a unique and frequently convoluted one, with each individual or couple experiencing their own set of problems. Understanding when to seek expert counsel on reproductive concerns is an important component of family planning since it ensures that possible problems are addressed quickly and efficiently. We go into many scenarios and concerns that signify the need for expert assistance in this thorough book, arming individuals and couples with the information to make informed decisions on their reproductive journey.

Age-Related Concerns: Timing Matters

Age is a critical aspect in determining whether to seek professional advice. If a woman over the age of 35 has been trying to conceive for six months or more without success, she should see a fertility specialist. For women under the age of 35, the timetable is extended to one year. Age has a substantial impact on fertility, and early intervention can be critical in resolving age-related issues.

Irregular Menstrual Cycles: How to Determine Ovulation

Irregular menstrual cycles might make finding the best time to conceive difficult. Women who are experiencing irregular cycles should seek professional help to investigate potential underlying causes and obtain advice on maximizing fertility in the setting of irregular cycles.

Previous Reproductive Health Issues: Preventative Measures

Individuals who have a history of reproductive health difficulties, such as polycystic ovary syndrome (PCOS) or endometriosis, should seek expert help as soon as possible.

Understanding how these illnesses may affect fertility, as well as receiving advice on appropriate interventions, is critical for informed family planning.

Known Male Factors: Understanding Sperm Health

Couples who are aware of male reproductive concerns, such as low sperm count or motility issues, should seek professional help right away. Early intervention can provide insights into probable reasons and appropriate treatment options for male reproductive health, which is an important component of fertility.

Multiple Miscarriages: Addressing Underlying Causes

Multiple losses can be emotionally draining and may indicate underlying reproductive concerns. Seeking expert help in such situations allows for a thorough review to discover relevant causes and establish a targeted plan for future efforts at conception.

Persistent Concerns: Addressing Apprehensions

Concerns about fertility, regardless of age or previous attempts, should be addressed by a specialist. Individuals or couples who are dealing with continuing issues or uncertainty can benefit from a complete evaluation by reproductive specialists to address concerns and explore viable solutions.

Pre-existing Medical Conditions: Considering Health Impacts

Individuals who have pre-existing medical illnesses, such as diabetes or thyroid issues, should seek expert help to determine how these conditions may affect fertility. Understanding the relationship between health and fertility is critical for building a comprehensive strategy for family planning.

Unprotected Intercourse: Timely Evaluation

Couples who engage in unprotected intercourse without conception for an extended period should seek expert help. A timely evaluation can assist in identifying probable variables contributing to reproductive issues and directing couples to the most effective next actions.

Occupational Exposures: Mitigating Risks

Those who are exposed to reproductive dangers at work, such as certain chemicals or radiation, should get help as soon as possible. Professional guidance can assist in assessing risks, making suggestions for reducing exposures, and addressing any effects on fertility.

Emotional Toll: Navigating the Journey

The emotional cost of infertility should not be underestimated. Seeking professional help early on can help individuals and couples navigate the emotional complexity that comes with fertility issues. Professionals in mental health play an important role in offering assistance and coping skills.

Knowledge Empowers Decisions Knowing when to seek expert counsel on reproductive issues is a powerful step in the route to parenting. This thorough handbook seeks to equip individuals and couples with the knowledge necessary to identify crucial indications and make timely and educated decisions. Seeking expert counsel, whether for age-related concerns, reproductive health difficulties, or mental well-being, establishes the groundwork for a proactive and supportive approach to family planning. Early intervention and coordination with fertility professionals help to boost the odds of successful conception and the achievement of the desire of children when negotiating the challenges of fertility.

The Crucial Role of Healthcare Professionals in Fertility: Nurturing Hope and Providing Guidance

Parenting is a meaningful and often challenging undertaking, and at its center is a collaborative partnership with reproductive specialists. Aside from diagnosis, these devoted personnel provide thorough care, emotional support, and individualized direction. In this in-depth examination, we dig into the numerous contributions of fertility healthcare specialists, putting light on their critical role in navigating the complex landscape of reproductive health.

Diagnostic Expertise: Unveiling the Complexity of Fertility Specialized Assessments

Fertility healthcare specialists bring a plethora of diagnostic experience to the table. They uncover the complexities of each individual's fertility landscape through careful tests that involve testing hormone levels, inspecting reproductive anatomy, and studying lifestyle factors.

Diagnosis Precision: Their ability to pinpoint particular disorders, such as irregular ovulation, hormone imbalances, or structural abnormalities, serves as the cornerstone for customized treatment approaches.

Personalized Treatment Plans: Crafting Care Tailored to Individuals Holistic Approach:

Recognizing the individuality of each reproductive journey, healthcare providers create tailored treatment programs that take an individual's medical history, lifestyle circumstances, and emotional well-being into account.

Professionals advise clients through various ART alternatives, such as in vitro fertilization (IVF), intrauterine insemination (IUI), and fertility drugs, for those who require further support.

Emotional Support: Navigating the Emotional Landscape of Fertility Challenges

Understanding the emotional toll of fertility issues, healthcare experts offer individuals and couples a caring space to share their concerns, anxieties, and hopes.

Collaboration with Mental Health Specialists: Working with mental health specialists is essential for promoting emotional well-being and resilience throughout the fertility journey.

Patient Education: Empowering Informed Choices

Transparent Communication: Healthcare professionals prioritize transparent communication to keep individuals and couples informed about their fertility status, potential challenges, and available options.

Empowering Decision-Making: They enable individuals to actively participate in decision-making through patient education, fostering a sense of control and ownership over their reproductive journey.

Monitoring and Adjustments: Adapting to Progress and Challenges

Healthcare specialists conduct regular assessments throughout the fertility treatment procedure to check progress and handle any emergent issues.

They tailor treatment approaches depending on individual reactions, increasing the likelihood of successful conception while limiting potential hazards.

Fertility Preservation: Planning for the Future

Individuals facing circumstances such as age, medical treatments, or job choices that may impair fertility are guided through fertility preservation options by healthcare specialists.

Strategic preparation: Future preparation, such as egg or sperm freezing, allows individuals to retain reproductive alternatives.

Preconception Counseling: Optimizing Conditions for Conception

Preconception counseling is provided by healthcare professionals, who advise on lifestyle variables that can affect fertility. This covers nutrition, exercise, and lifestyle guidelines to improve reproductive health.

Recognizing and Addressing Potential Risk Factors: Recognizing and addressing potential risk factors, helps to create an optimal environment for conception and a safe pregnancy.

Advocacy and Empowerment: Navigating Difficult Decisions

Patient Advocacy: Healthcare professionals act as advocates for their patients, negotiating difficult decisions and organizing care with a multidisciplinary team.

Individual Empowerment: Through advocacy and support, they enable individuals to persevere in the face of adversity, building a sense of resilience and resolve.

The work of fertility healthcare professionals extends beyond the clinical sphere; it is a tapestry stitched with competence, sensitivity, and unwavering dedication. These specialists aid individuals and couples on the path to motherhood by unraveling the complexity of reproductive health, delivering tailored care, and giving emotional support. Their numerous contributions not only increase the likelihood of successful conception, but also foster optimism, resilience, and the fulfillment of the dream of starting a family. The song of possibility is performed in the collaborative dance between healthcare professionals and aspiring parents, mirroring the promise of new beginnings and the fulfillment of long-held hopes.

Conclusion

Nourishing the Journey to Fertility with Boost Smoothies

As we navigate the complex landscape of fertility, finding answers and embracing holistic approaches becomes critical. In the course of this journey, fertility-boosting smoothies emerge as more than just a tasty concoction of flavors, but also as a potent elixir that nourishes both the body and the spirit. Our research into fertility boost smoothies for couples has shown a tapestry of flavors, nutrients, and lifestyle changes that have the promise of improving reproductive health.

A Symphony of Nutrients: The Building Blocks of Fertility

The fertility boost smoothies given are a symphony of well-chosen ingredients, each of which contributes its melody to the overall composition. These smoothies are designed to target various areas of reproductive health, from antioxidant-rich berries to fertility-boosting walnuts and hormone-regulating maca powder. Couples go on a journey where nutrition becomes a vital component in the orchestration of fertility by harnessing the power of nature's bounty.

Lifestyle Harmony: Beyond the Blender

However, the benefits of fertility booster smoothies go beyond the contents. It interacts with lifestyle choices, encouraging couples to adopt practices that promote overall well-being. Regular physical exercise, stress management, and proper sleep work in tandem with these smoothies to supply a comprehensive approach to the varied aspects of fertility.

From Sam and Sarah to Every Couple: A Blueprint for Hope

The story of Sam and Sarah, our fictional couple on a reproductive journey, serves as a model for many others who are treading similar ground. Their hardships and achievements echo the universal struggles and hopes buried in the fertility journey. We see the transforming impact of nutrition, lifestyle changes, and emotional support in shaping the fertility landscape through the lens of their story.

Empowerment through Knowledge: A Key to Fertility Success

The road to fertility is frequently fraught with uncertainties and questions. However, we may view the empowerment

that comes with knowledge through the lens of fertility boost smoothies. Couples who understand the nutrients that promote reproductive health and the lifestyle choices that can improve fertility are better prepared to face any issues that may emerge.

The Role of Communication: A Vital Component of Fertility Wellness

Communication, both with one another and with healthcare providers, emerges as an essential component of fertility wellness. The candor of Sam and Sarah about their worries, shared decision-making, and collaboration with healthcare experts demonstrate the importance of creating a supportive atmosphere. This underscores the larger truth that seeking expert help, particularly when dealing with fertility issues, is a proactive step toward a more educated and guided path.

Diversity in Fertility: A Tapestry of Stories

It's critical to recognize that fertility is as unique as the people and couples that experience it. While fertility boost smoothies can be a tasty and nutritious complement to your journey, there is no one-size-fits-all approach. Each individual's experience is unique and impacted by a variety of factors such as genetics, lifestyle, and medical history. Fertility is thus a tapestry of stories, each with its own set of struggles, perseverance, and achievements.

A Call to Holistic Fertility Care: Integrating Approaches

We advocate for an integrated and holistic approach to fertility care as we conclude our investigation on fertility-boosting smoothies. A holistic strategy is built on the synergy of diet, lifestyle choices, emotional well-being, and expert supervision. Fertility is a dynamic interaction of physical, emotional, and environmental elements, and addressing it necessitates a multidimensional approach that understands and respects the human body's and reproductive system's complexity.

Hope, Resilience, and the Fertility Journey

In essence, the fertility journey is a story of hope and perseverance. It's a trip that tests, transforms, and eventually promises fresh beginnings. conception boost smoothies, with their brilliant hues and nutrient-rich formulations, represent a commitment to nourishing the body and mind to boost conception. They serve as a reminder that, even in the face of uncertainty, there are concrete steps individuals and couples may take to improve their reproductive health.

The Uncharted Future: Navigating with Optimism

As we come to the end of our exploration of fertility booster smoothies, we acknowledge that the future is unknown, with twists and turns that may surprise or challenge us. Couples engage on this path with optimism, armed with knowledge, reinforced by support networks, and enjoying the nourishing power of fertility boost smoothies. The symphony of nutrients, the harmony of lifestyle choices, and the tenacity of the human spirit all come together to form a melody that guides each couple on their path to fatherhood. May this tune bring you to hope, health, and the fulfillment of your dream of starting a family.